The Genius of Ordinary Food

The evolutionary journey of a single-cell amoeba to a 37.2 trillion cell human being.

By Matt Wright

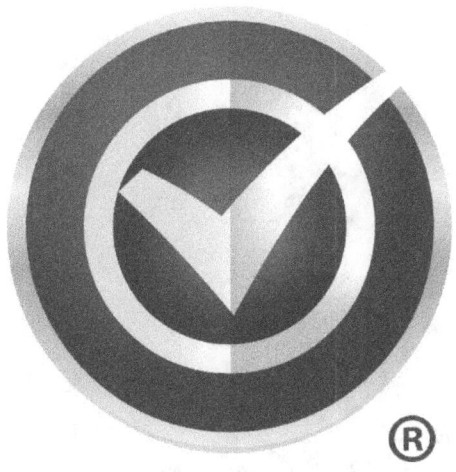

Published by Check Your Food Ltd
Brighton UK

The information provided in this book has been carefully considered and checked by the author. It should not, however, be regarded as a substitute for competent medical advice. Therefore all information in this book is provided without any warranty or guarantee on the part of the author or publisher. Neither the author nor the publisher or their representatives shall bear any liability whatsoever for personal injury, property damage, and financial losses.

Contents

"From spirulina to goji berries, from fat free to sugar free, from vitamin supplements to skin creams, from cholesterol lowering drugs to anti-depressants. The array of options for the health-conscious consumer to consider are endless.

Why not stop for a minute and take note of what our ordinary daily food can do for us?"
Matt Wright - Author

Preface

"I would not exist if it wasn't for chickens' feet!"

This book has come from a 45 year fascination with food. This fascination started when I was 8 years old and my dad dropped a chicken's foot on my dinner plate and said "Eat that son, you wouldn't exist if it wasn't for chickens' feet."

The story behind the chickens' feet....

In 1929, my dad and his identical twin brother were born in a small house in east London. Unfortunately, a few months later they both contracted severe whooping cough and could not hold any food down. My grandfather was told that there was nothing the doctors could do and that the twins should be left to die. Now my grandfather was a Billingsgate fishmonger and he had a friend in the chicken business who told him to try 'chicken's foot jelly'. This is obtained by boiling chickens' feet and letting the resulting liquid cool into a jelly. Guess what, this turned out to be the only food the twins could hold down. They dealt with the bacterial infection and as a consequence they both survived and went on to lead healthy lives.

And of course one of them became my dad!

Many of us love and enjoy food but are largely unaware of the myriad of benefits that food gives to our bodies and our environment.

I want to inspire you to take even more pleasure and delight in what you eat, secure in the knowledge of the amazing power food has to keep you alive - yes, but also to enhance, invigorate and push you to levels of health, happiness and energy you may have only dreamt about.

Various foods will 'enter' the book, with one or two nutrients being highlighted from each one. I leave the discovery of all the other goodness I have left out to your further research.

I have made the assumption that the macronutrients of fats, protein and carbohydrate are in almost every ingredient we look at. However, the ingenuity I am focussing on comes from the smaller nutrients found in food, known as 'micronutrients'.

Whilst a lot of science and history will be referenced, I won't be covering the findings of every study, observation and record. Everything I say and allude to in this book has its origins in the accepted biological, chemical and physical sciences, along with various historical findings and records. The book also contains a bit of creative licence thrown in for the purposes of illustration.

Creative licence

This book follows the evolution of 'Eva' from a single-cell amoeba to a fully developed multi-cellular organism (such as we are), via the food she eats along her evolutionary path. This story is of course a fable and thus will lack exact archaeological, anatomical and digestive accuracy. However, the contributions made to Eva's development by the various foods are based in sound science. For every meat ingredient I subsequently give a **vEva** (vegetarian Eva) equivalent with the same genius.

Around 3,500 million years ago, life consisted primarily of single prokaryotic cells (cells without a nucleus). Somewhere along the line, these cells turned eukaryotic (developed a nucleus), banded together and began to form single coherent organisms. This 'banding together' may have taken a billion years or so.

Scientists refer to this time as the 'boring billion' as from an evolutionary point of view, nothing much of interest happened.

Or did it?

Meet Eva

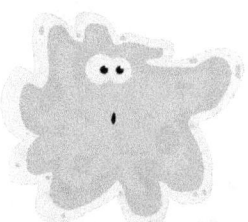

This is Eva, a single-cell amoeba. What sets her apart from her fellow single-cell creatures is her insatiable appetite. Eva was so hungry and greedy, it eventually led to her Dad asking her to leave her little community.

"You're too greedy!"

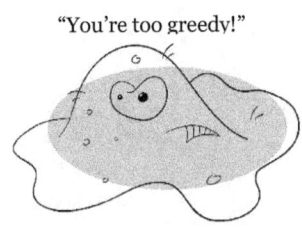

Eva - who was tired of her single-cell existence - welcomed this opportunity to leave her friends in order to find more food, and hopefully a new and exciting anatomy...

Chapter One

Cells and DNA

An amoeba close up

Amoeba = a single-cell organism.

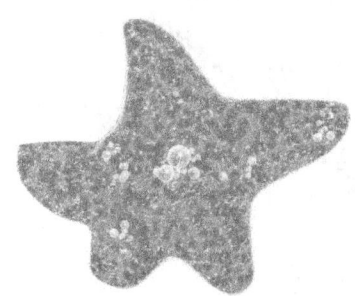

Human zygote (first stage of life at fertilisation of the egg) = a single-cell organism.

Fully developed Human Being = a self-repairing organism made up of 37.2 trillion cells (latest estimate).

A cell close up

"All the processes necessary for life can take place in a single cell."
UK Open University - Cells and Nutrition

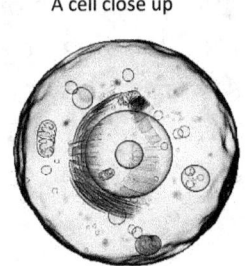

Every minute, 96 million of our cells die and 96 million new ones are made.

"DNA is like a computer program but far, far more advanced than any software ever created."
Bill Gates

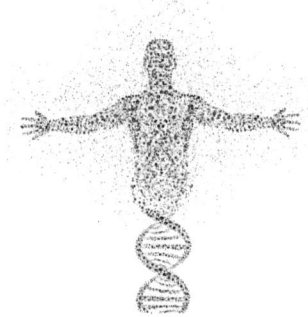

Eva, some science, history and a lot of eating...

And so Eva left home and immediately set about finding something to eat. And as she was rolling along, she stumbled over something that had just fallen out of a tree and hit the ground. Bending down to take a closer look, she saw a small hard lump." Whatever can this be?" thought Eva, "And more importantly: can I eat it?"

Enter the Hazelnut

The hazelnut was being cultivated over 9,000 years ago. This classic nut can be eaten raw, roasted, or made into flour or a paste for use in baking. Traditionally, this nut was roasted to extend its shelf life, especially for use by mariners.

Today 20 cultivated types of hazelnut are grown in Europe, Turkey, Iran, India, and the US. The global supply is over 780,000 tons, 25% of which are used to make Nutella, the famous chocolate spread!

The hazelnut delivers a powerful nutrient that helps our DNA create new cells - a handy nutrient for a hungry single-cell organism looking for a new anatomy!

Eva crunched down the nut, swallowed with a large gulp and found herself with the necessary resources to create more DNA and cells from the vitamin **Biotin** (also known as vitamin B7).

*Biotin plays a role in the healthy activity of our cells and DNA regulation; it also regulates inflammation and protects the development of babies.

Despite being armed with a sack of hazelnuts, Eva was even more ravenous now. And so she set off to find her next meal. In the distance, Eva spotted a mass of green shapes. "Great! These have got to be edible!" she thought.

Enter the Spinach Leaf

Spinach (made famous by Popeye, at least the tinned version), is native to central and western Asia and thought to have originated in Persia.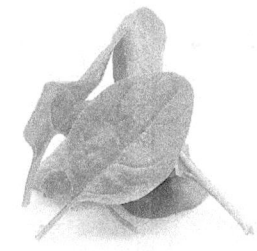
When introduced to ancient China, it was known as the "Persian vegetable".

Spinach eventually reached Europe in the 9th century, when the Saracens brought it to Sicily. One "spinach myth" is that Popeye's legendary strength came from a misplaced decimal point in the amount of iron spinach contained, crediting spinach with 10 times the actual iron it contains.

It has since been claimed that spinach gave Popeye super strength because of its carotene content. However, for Eva's development we are focused on a different nutrient that spinach is a great source of.

This amazing leaf delivers a nutrient that is essential for DNA creation and ongoing repair and is vital for the creation and maintenance of new cells. Very necessary for an organism whose cell is looking to divide and duplicate!

Eva gobbled up the green leaves, and from the vitamin **Folate** (also known as vitamin B9) in the spinach now had even more resources to create healthy cells.

*Folate prevents birth defects, is essential for DNA creation and repair, lowers the risk of heart disease and cancer, regulates inflammation, and is essential for normal brain function.

Eva, still ravenous, went on her way in search of more food and soon ran into 3 new friends...

Enter the Eggs

"Well hello!" thought Eva whilst sizing up their potential edibility. The eggs - who had been on a bit of a 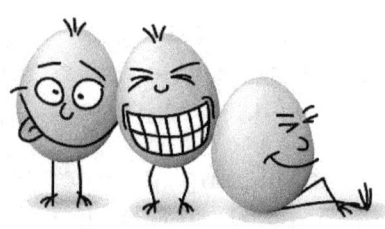 lunchtime session - giggled as they pushed each other around. Finally, after much jovial pushing and shoving, one of them toppled over and broke, releasing the albumen and yolk. "Oh, wow!" thought Eva "Food!" She swooped on the gloopy fluid, slurping it all up, before and sitting down with a bump, belching loudly. The other 2 eggs looked on a little sadly and went on their way.

Eggs from domesticated chickens are said to have originated in China and India over 7,000 years ago, and have likely been eaten by us for a lot longer, due the ease with which they can be gathered (eggs don't bite). An estimated 62 million tons of chicken eggs are produced a year, from 6.4 billion egg laying hens. The European Union has recently banned the battery farming of chickens to produce eggs and meat, thanks to the likes of Hugh Fearnley-Whittingstall.

The incredible egg provides us with the most complex of nutrients, which is essential for DNA and cell replication and - along with the folate from spinach - prevents birth defects.

With the **Vitamin B12** from the egg, Eva now had nearly all the resources for her cell replication and division - but she still was starving for more food.

*Vitamin B12 is essential for the healthy duplication of DNA, works with folate to decrease the risk of birth defects, and with vitamin B6 to decrease our risk of heart disease and cancer.

Continuing on her journey, Eva entered a waterlogged field and noticed some very tasty looking plants in the sludge...

Enter the grass we call Rice

Chinese legend has it that rice production was originated by Shennong, a legendary emperor of China, his name meaning the 'Divine Farmer'. Genetic evidence has shown that rice originated from a single domestication up to 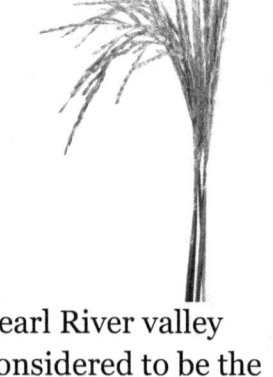 13,500 years ago in the Pearl River valley region of China. Rice is considered to be the most important grain for human nutrition, providing more than one-fifth of the calories consumed by humans worldwide.

In its less refined form (brown), this great grain gives us two nutrients that are essential for the creation and repair of DNA, as well as turning fats and carbs into energy.

Eva pounced on the rice and ate it raw (not advisable) and had to stop as it began to swell inside her at an alarming rate (when cooked, rice expands to up to 3 times its original size).

Once she had recovered, Eva - now equipped with the mineral **Magnesium** and the vitamin **Niacin** (also known as vitamin B3) - was nearly fully prepared for expansion but still had some more nutrients to encounter before entering the next phase of her life.

Magnesium turns fats and carbs into cellular energy, plays a role in the creation of antioxidants and is essential for the creation of DNA.

Niacin enables our cells to "talk" to each other to keep us healthy, plays a vital role in our energy production and may play a significant role in the prevention of cancer.

Eva continued on her journey and noticed a plant with green dangly bits. Opening one up, she noticed a very comfortable looking fur lining with small green objects nestling in it. "These definitely look delicious!" thought our greedy Eva.

Enter the Broad Bean

Remains of broad
beans have been
found in the
Egyptian tombs,
and spread to
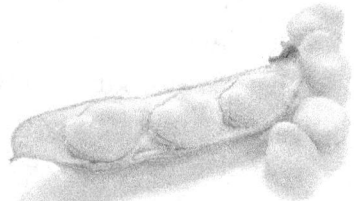
Northern Italy during the Bronze Age (4,300
years ago). Ancient remains of broad beans
have been found at Glastonbury in the UK -
and due to their detoxification properties
probably still come in handy at a certain time
of the year.

Broad beans are very easy to grow, survive
winter, and – importantly - they fix nitrogen in
the soil, an essential process for all forms of
life.

The broad bean is rich in a nutrient that keeps
our cells in good order, turns food into energy
and enables our liver to deal with toxins.

Eva proceeded to bolt as many of these green
objects as she could, if a little more cautiously
than before (due to her swelling experience
with the rice).

Now full of the vitamin **Pantothenic Acid**
(also known as vitamin B5), Eva had more
resources for healthy cell division, along with

energy creation and the ability to deal with any toxins she may encounter along the way.

Pantothenic acid enables our liver to cope with toxins, plays a vital role in generating energy from our food and keeps our cells in good order.

Still very hungry, Eva noticed an odd smell emanating from a yellow blob on the ground. "Smell or no smell, I *have* to try this!" she thought. To Eva, everything had the potential to be edible, not unlike a human baby.

Enter the Cheeses

The history of cheese predates recorded history, so dates back more than 8,000 years: in his Odyssey, Homer described Cyclops as a cheesemaker.

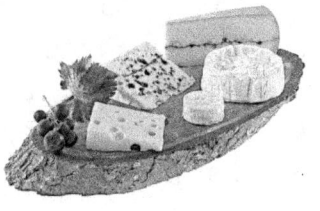

The earliest cheeses were most likely similar to modern cottage cheese and feta, with the heavy use of salt preserving this dairy product.

In the UK during World War II, artisan cheese making was banned by the government, and all cheese makers were instructed to only produce mild cheddar to keep the rationed population supplied with this rich source of nutrients. This led to the distinct advantage the French had in the production of artisan cheeses, which survived until the recent revival of UK cheese.

As has been said before: 'blessed are the cheese makers', for this ingredient yields a whole host of supporting factors for a developing organism.

Along with many other good things, cheese is full of a nutrient that is used by every cell in our bodies to work normally.

Eva swooped down on the cheese and enjoyed it's salty, savoury tanginess (a flavour combination found in a mature cheddar-type of cheese), and now, packed with the mineral **Phosphorus,** was even more ready for the next phase of her life**.**

*Phosphorus is required by every cell in our bodies to work normally; it is critical in creating our energy and maintaining the chemical balance of our bodies.

The ever-hungry Eva was now ready for another meal - and lo and behold, a shiny looking thing came rolling down the hill, conveniently coming to rest at her feet. Looking down, Eva thought "Oh, how am I going to eat this?"

Enter the Baked Beans

Tinned baked beans are made from the haricot or navy bean and stewed in a tomato sauce. This popular staple 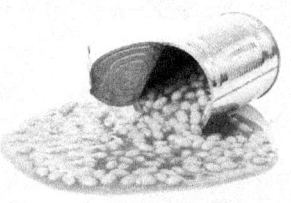 originated in America and first came to the UK in 1886.

Baked beans can be eaten straight from the tin as they are pre-cooked. First, the dried beans are boiled, then baked in tomato sauce at a low temperature for several hours to allow the flavours to infuse the beans.

Baked beans contain a fantastic nutrient that supports our DNA and energy creation, and protects our eyes.

Eva took on the challenge, and after hitting the tin repeatedly with a rock, she managed to split it and gorge on the contents. Now equipped with the vitamin **Thiamin** (also known as vitamin B1), Eva was finally ready for the next phase of her life, but decided she needed just one more meal...

Whilst eating the beans, Eva had spotted a bright red thing at the side of the road that looked very tempting. Bending down, she picked up this intriguing soft lump and popped it into her mouth. "Heavenly," thought Eva.

Enter the Strawberry

Interestingly, the strawberry is first mentioned in ancient Roman literature as a medicine. It is the French who are credited with taking the wild strawberry from the forest and domesticating it in the 14th century. The strawberries-and-cream dish made so famous by the Wimbledon Tennis Tournament was created at the court of King Henry the VIII by Thomas Wolsey (the famous cardinal).

The common strawberry we have today came from North America to Europe in the 17th century, with only the female plants bearing this summer favourite.

The strawberry contains a group of chemicals (known as phytochemicals) that the berry uses to protect itself from disease, and eating strawberries passes on this protection to us. Phytochemicals provide protection for our DNA and cell replication by keeping our cells communicating clearly with each other.

Cell communication or 'signalling' - definition

The ability of cells to perceive and correctly respond to their microenvironment is the basis of development, tissue repair, and immunity. Errors in cell communication are responsible for diseases such as cancer, autoimmunity, and diabetes.

Loving the sweetness of the red berries, Eva guzzled them down until all of a sudden, full of the **Phytochemicals** from the strawberries, she began to change...

*Diets high in phytochemicals lead to a considerable reduction in the risk of heart disease, stroke, high blood pressure, cancer, osteoporosis and cataracts, and may be neuroprotective.

About cells

The latest estimate is that we have over 37 trillion cells that make us up, with about 200 hundred different types of cells.

We lose around 96 million cells a minute with 96 million new cells being made in that same minute!

Cell communication joke:

There were three old cells at a bus stop, the first one says "Is it windy today?"

The second cell replies "Oh, no, I think its Thursday."

To which the third cell chips in "Oooh so am I, let's have a cup of tea."

Some cell types

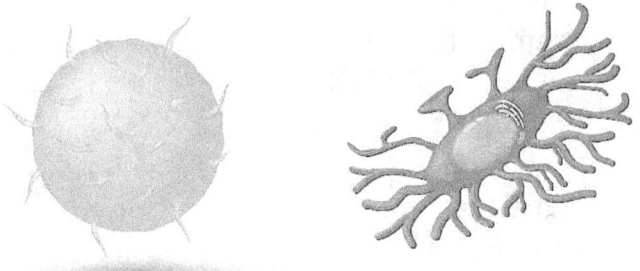

Blood cell

Bone cell

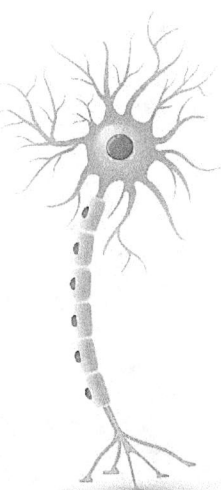

Motor neurone cell

Summary

Nutrients critical to cell and DNA health

1. Biotin (B7)
2. Folate (B9)
3. Vitamin B12
4. Pantothenic acid (B5)
5. Thiamin (B1)
6. Niacin (B3)
7. Magnesium
8. Phosphorus
9. Phytochemicals

A cell dividing

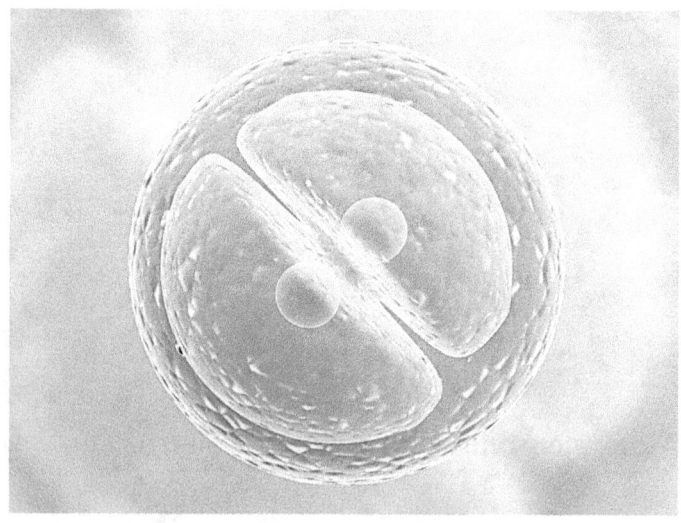

Chapter Two

The Immune System

"Whenever the immune system deals successfully with an infection, it emerges from the experience stronger and better able to confront similar threats in the future. Our immune system develops in combat. If, at the first sign of infection, you always jump in with antibiotics, you do not give the immune system a chance to grow stronger."
Andrew Weil - MD

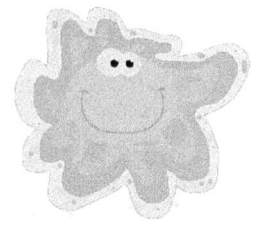 Eva, now equipped with new cells (and a smile) from her binge-eating of hazelnuts, spinach, eggs, raw rice (much better for you when cooked), broad beans, cheese, baked beans and strawberries, continued on her way.

Soon she reached a crossroads with 3 signposts. One said "Plant Kingdom" (green and edible), one said "Fungus Kingdom" (mouldy and damp), and the last one said "Animal Kingdom" (arms, legs and self-awareness). "Hmmm," thought Eva, "which one to take?"

Eva sat down to eat another strawberry and tried to think (very difficult without a brain!). Eventually she came to the conclusion that the idea of arms, legs and self-awareness sounded best, so she picked up her sack of supplies and set off down the Animal Kingdom road.

Around 2,000 million years ago, the Eukaryote life domain was a collection of 'true cells' - that is cells with a nucleus - and these cells went down one of the three paths: plant, fungus or animal.

Eva continued down the Animal Kingdom road for a while, until she heard a noise in the distance...

Eva goes to a Party

In a clearing, a group of very odd looking creatures were jostling, all slobbering over each other and gnashing their teeth, whilst loud music was playing.

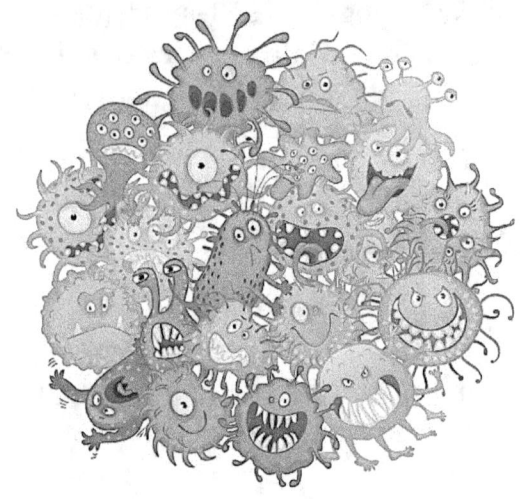

"Wow, I would love a set of those!" thought Eva, temporarily forgetting her hunger.

"Hey, come and join us!" shouted a bright green blob.

"Do you have anything to eat?" Eva yelled back.

"Oh boy, do we!" chuckled the bright green blob.

"Well…" thought Eva "what could possibly go wrong?"

The bright green blob introduced himself as H5NI and proceeded to introduce Eva to Pertussis, Salmonella, H1N1, Herpes Simplex and his sister Varicella, streptococcus, and lastly lactobacillus. "What a collection!" thought Eva, immediately taking a dislike to all of them except Lactobacillus, and with good reason...

Enter the Viruses & Bacteria

Bacteria are a 3,500 million year old domain of life made up of some particularly nasty types like Pertussis (whooping cough), mixed in with some very positive and giving types such as lactobacillus, which enhance our digestive system.

Viruses are not classified as life and their origins are not entirely clear. However, they are very real and pose both an advantage and a threat to a developing organism. The H5N1 is a bird flu virus with very nasty and potentially fatal effects on humans; however, the HER-V virus group has injected its genetic material into the human genome. We exist as modern humans in part due to the HER-V virus group!

Eva joined the party and noticed that everyone kept brushing up against her and giggling. "Whatever are they trying to do?" she thought.

As there was nothing to eat at this party, Eva soon said her goodbyes. As she moved on down the road, she began to feel a little strange...

"I do feel most odd..." thought Eva.

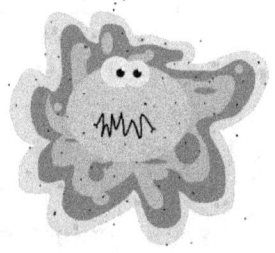

Unfortunately, Eva had contracted a bacterial infection, namely Pertussis (whooping cough), and a virus, namely H5N1 or bird flu, "Oh dear, whatever shall I do now?" thought Eva.

Luckily she had also picked up some positive digestive assistance from lactobacillus, and still very hungry, she spotted a long yellow object hanging from a huge plant by the side of the road...

Enter the Banana

Bananas are said to have been first cultivated in New Guinea around 10,000 years ago. From there, they 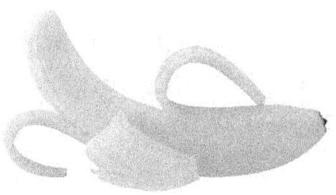 spread to the Philippines and then across the tropics. Bananas are naturally radioactive and are sometimes used to compare radiation levels, based on what is known as the 'Banana unit'.

Strictly speaking, the banana is not a tree fruit but a 'herb', and in Britain we eat over 5 billion bananas a year (at an average of 2 per week per person).

The banana is often referred to as a 'high herb', partly due to the height it grows at and also perhaps as a reference to the teenage practice of drying out the skins and smoking them.

The herby banana contains a nutrient that enables us to deal with viruses and bacteria by providing support for our immune system. The banana is not famous for this particular nutrient - a nutrient that is vital for our immune system and also helps transporting oxygen around our bodies and keeping us happy.

Eva scoffed the banana (once she worked out how to peel it) and, as a result of the effects of the **Vitamin B6**, began to feel a little better.

*Vitamin B6 maintains our immune system, keeps us happy, helps oxygen circulating throughout our bodies and reduces our risk of heart disease.

Despite now being the owner of the beginnings of an immune system, Eva was still feeling decidedly unwell, and yet she wanted more food. At this point, she stumbled over a curved red lump. "Wow!" thought Eva "This looks yummy!"

Enter the Lamb Cutlet

The lamb cutlet is a cut from just behind the neck and is often served in a 'rack'. Lamb is a domestic sheep of around 1 year of age. According to the Bible, God is partial to lamb served whole and charred (see Leviticus 1:3 on burnt offerings).

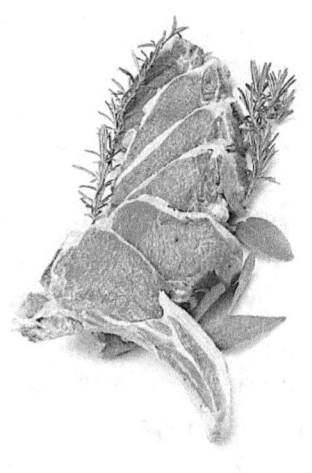

Lamb cutlets or chops can be fried, grilled or roasted. The French have a habit of trimming off all the best bits and serving lamb cutlets with a bone ("French-trimmed") that has had all the flavour removed, but then again what do the French know about cooking?

Lamb is always free range and is served with what is known as "tracklements" - herbs such as rosemary and mint that the lamb would have eaten naturally in its short life.

Lamb fat has now been found to have distinct health benefits due to its grass and forage (herbs and weeds) diet, but more on that later.

Lamb meat contains three nutrients that are essential for the proper functioning of our immune system - and very much needed by Eva to deal with the whooping cough and bird flu.

In addition to supporting our immune system, these nutrients also regulate our moods and sleep, remove the toxic effects of heavy metals, and help us to absorb the goodness of folate (think the spinach Eva ate earlier).

Eva chowed down on the cutlet, and from the action of the **Zinc** and the essential amino acids **Tryptophan** and **Histidine** began to feel even better.

Zinc is an essential mineral for our immune system, growth and development, brain function, reproduction and skin health.

Tryptophan helps our immune system, regulates our moods and sleep and can reduce anxiety and depression.

Histidine regulates our immune system and has a cleansing role in the body.

The fat of lamb has been very unpopular in recent years, with all sorts of negative claims being made. I will leave those arguments to one side and mention **Conjugated Linoleic Acid,** a natural trans-fat present in lamb (as opposed to the nasty stuff created by processing sub-par vegetable oils). Conjugated linoleic acid or CLA has anti-cancer properties, a fact that was discovered "by accident" in a laboratory.

Conjugated linoleic acid is a fatty acid that has been shown to have powerful anti-cancer properties.

The **vEva** equivalents – Cheese, Eggs, Peanuts

Eva, now equipped with a steadily improving immune system, spotted the top of a bright orange object poking out of the ground. As she was still very hungry, Eva pounced on it, pulled it up and thought "Now this looks decidedly appetising."

Enter the Carrot

Our familiar orange carrot is a descendant of the wild purple carrot, seeds for which have been discovered in Europe from 5,000 years ago. Carrot cultivation is believed to have originated in Afghanistan, with the orange carrot coming 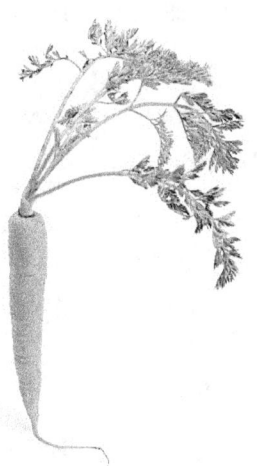 from Turkey and later being refined in Holland (in the 16th century), giving us our modern sweet orange carrot.

The dazzling carrot contains a group of chemicals that contribute to the health of our heart, provide protection from cancer and can be transformed by us into an even more potent nutrient that boosts our immune system, repairs our cells and protects our sight.

Eva studied the carrot for a while and thought "This looks tough to chew, if only there was a way to soften it."

Nevertheless, Eva proceeded to scarf down this tough little root. Luckily Eva washed the carrot down with some nuts which made it even easier for her developing body to absorb all its goodness.

Fat and carrots:
carrots on their own = pass through
carrots + fat (from the nuts) = absorbed

The cooking and the softening of carrots:
The goodness in carrots is made much more available to us if we cook them lightly to break down the tough structure and release the life-enhancing chemicals.

Due to the **Carotenes** in the carrot, some of which had converted to **Vitamin A** in Eva, her immune system had become even stronger.

*Vitamin A is vital in protecting our bodies from infection and is a powerful antioxidant (cleanser/repairer).

Feeling very much better, Eva continued on her way and soon smelt something that was sure to be delicious as she came across a pot bubbling by the side of the road. "How convenient" thought Eva, "I wonder what this might be?" Lifting the lid, Eva saw some brown lumps gently simmering in a pool of liquid, surrounded by those lovely carrots again. Eva dived straight in to the pot (don't try this at home) and devoured the whole lot in 3 gulps.

Enter the grass-fed Beef Brisket

The beef brisket is a cut from the lower chest of a cow and comes from the muscles that support 60% of the animal's 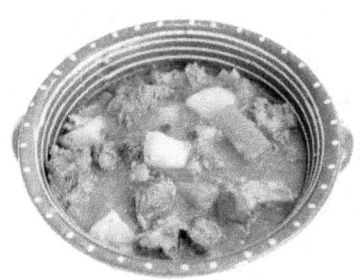 weight making it very tough. This is why it benefits from slow cooking.

The beef brisket features in many World Cuisines, including Jewish, Chinese, Korean, Thai, British, Italian and Indian. In recent 'Man versus Food' times, brisket is perhaps best known as a classic American dish served smoked, braised and cured into corned beef.

Brisket contains, amongst many others, 2 more essential nutrients required for the full functioning of our immune system, and both specifically target viruses. These two are also involved in the various cleansing and repairing mechanisms so vital to our long-term health.

Having recovered from her first bath in a stew, Eva was now benefiting from the minerals **Iron** and **Selenium** and nearly had a complete defence system against the pertussis and H5N1.

*Selenium regenerates the activity of vitamins C and E, produces several antioxidants (cleansers & repairers) and enhances our immune system.

*Iron is vital for enabling our immune system to kill viruses and bacteria, and for the transport of oxygen around our body.

Grass-fed beef is also a good source of **Conjugated Linoleic Acid,** making this popular cut even more beneficial for us.

*The **vEva** equivalent – Brazil Nuts, Jerusalem Artichokes*

Still ravenous, Eva thought: "Hmmm what next - perhaps something sweet?" And just as she was thinking this, she noticed a tree with bright orbs hanging from it. "Now these have got to be good!" thought Eva, getting excited at the prospect of even more eating.

Enter the Orange

The orange is a
hybrid between the
pomelo and the
mandarin, being
made up of 25%
pomelo genes and
75% mandarin genes.
Sweet oranges are

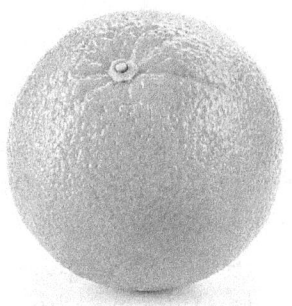

mentioned in Chinese literature as long as
2,500 years ago and are now the most
cultivated fruit in the world. Over 71 million
tons of oranges are grown each year, mainly in
Spain, Brazil, Florida and California. Navel
oranges are so named because they have a spot
on them that very closely resembles the human
belly button.

Dressed in its thick skin, the resplendent
orange offers a nutrient that everyone is
familiar with and that keeps our immune
system in tip top shape. It is also critical for
brain function (a later stage in Eva's
development).

Eva ate the orange whole (a nutritious if bitter
way to enjoy an orange), and from the surge of
Vitamin C now had an even more complete

set of the nutrients so vital for her defence against that party hangover.

Vitamin C keeps our immune system in tip top shape and is a very powerful antioxidant (cleanser/repairer).

Feeling almost whole again, Eva sensed she needed a couple more things to set her completely straight and finally rid herself of those two interlopers from the party that had tried to take over her system. "Now what is this grubby looking object that has just popped out of the ground?" thought Eva, "Let's eat it and find out what it does."

Enter the Mushroom

According to hieroglyphics from 4,600 years ago, the ancient Egyptians believed that the mushroom was the plant of immortality.

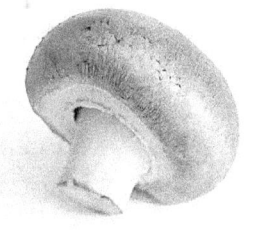

So revered was the mushroom that the pharaohs declared it to be only suitable for royalty. I can only assume that the swan must have similar properties in the UK?

Mushrooms are very easy to cultivate and generally packaged in attractive punnets. These were originally intended to attract more customers to what can be - let's face it - not a very alluring product.

The mushroom in its many forms offers an unfamiliar nutrient that is known to be very important for the development and maintenance of our immune system, along with helping our brain and nervous system.

Eva, having wolfed down the raw mushroom (not a bad idea as mushrooms are delicious raw), began to benefit from the mineral **Copper** and was now even closer to a fully functioning immune system.

Copper maintains our immune system and contributes to the cleansing and repairing activity of antioxidants.

Suddenly Eva had a yen for some more hazelnuts. Reaching into her knapsack, she pulled out a handful that she had cleverly shelled earlier on her journey and crunched them down.

Re-enter the Hazelnut

Along with the DNA support the hazelnut offers, this auspicious nut also provides two more nutrients that

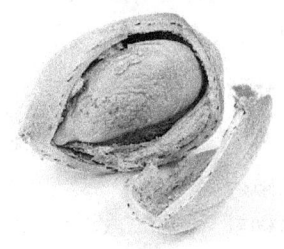

ensure a healthy immune system.

With the **Vitamin E** and the phytochemicals known as **Phytosterols** from the hazelnut, Eva now had almost everything required for a healthy immune system. She just needed one more (absolutely free and available on an almost daily basis) nutrient that would be the death knell for the pertussis and H5N1.

*Vitamin E keeps our immune system and skin healthy along with being a very powerful antioxidant.

*Phytosterols help our immune system stay healthy and maintain the positive activity of our cells.

Enter the Sun

The sun produces around 386 billion Megawatts of power and makes up 99.8% of the total mass in our solar system.

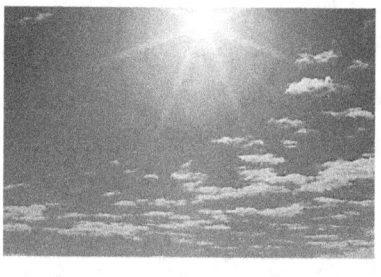

Around 1 million Earths would be able to fit into the sun!

With the arrival of the Mediterranean holiday in the 1960s, the glamour of sunbathing took off in the UK, too. In addition to making people turn brown, browner or just red for some of us, the sun has a powerful nutrient to offer us that is vital for our health.

The effect of the sun's rays on our skin enables us to produce a nutrient that enhances our immunity, along with being essential for our bones and nervous system.

Just 10 minutes of sunshine on bare skin 3 times a week between the hours of 11 and 2 p.m. from April to October can give us enough **Vitamin D** to last us the whole year, but only without sun cream (take note, parents).
Specified by Dr Michael Holick

Vitamin D enhances our immunity, is essential for our bone growth/maintenance, is vital for our nervous system, and protects against cancer.

After a whole lot of eating and a touch of sunbathing, Eva finally had a fully functioning immune system to protect her new-found cells.

And due to the incredible adaptive nature of our immune system, Eva now had lifelong protection from those strands of pertussis and H5N1.

That touch of sunbathing had made Eva hungry again. "It must be time for some more eating!" she thought as she began to change again...

The two systems

We have two immune systems, the 'innate' that provides immediate protection from bacteria and viruses with skin, sweat and mucus, and the 'adaptive' system. The adaptive system is the one that, having dealt with a virus or bacteria once, never forgets what they look like and will attack and destroy any future infections. The vaccinations that have wiped out major diseases like smallpox, polio and rubella trigger the genius of this adaptive system.

History of the Development of Medicine

Complaint: I have an earache.

2000 B.C: Eat this root

1000 A.D.: That root is heathen, say this prayer.

1850 A.D.: That prayer is superstition, drink this potion.

1940 A.D.: That potion is snake oil, swallow this pill.

1985 A.D.: That pill is ineffective, take this antibiotic.

2016 A.D.: That antibiotic is artificial. Here, eat this root.

A couple of immune system cells

Macrophage means 'big eater' in Greek, and these white blood cells are the first on the scene of an infection to 'engulf' viruses and bacteria.

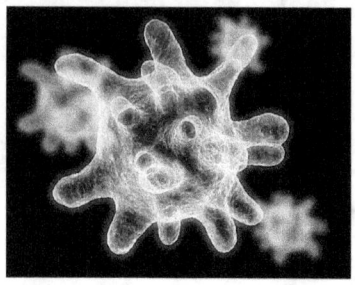

An isolated macrophage

The T cell is a highly specialised defender cell that is programmed to recognise an exact pathogen and destroy it.

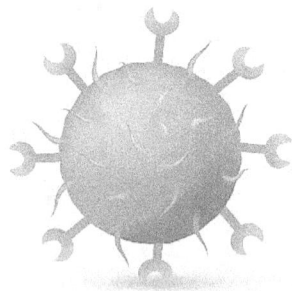

An isolated T cell

Summary

Nutrients critical to the health of our immune system

1. Vitamin B6
2. Zinc
3. Tryptophan
4. Histidine
5. Carotenes
6. Vitamin A
7. Selenium
8. Vitamin C
9. Copper
10. Vitamin E
11. Phytosterols
12. Vitamin D

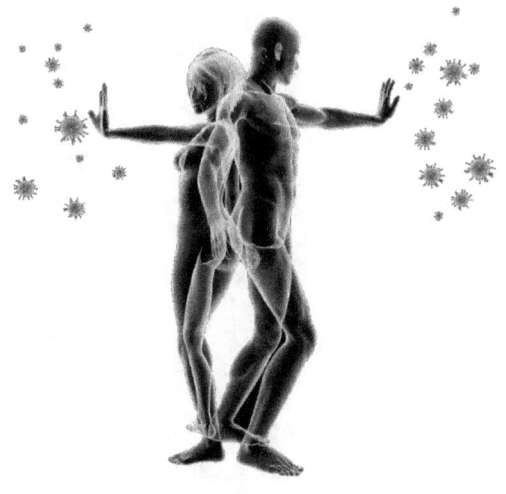

Chapter Three

Bones and Teeth

"The evil that men do lives after them; the good is oft interred with their bones."
William Shakespeare

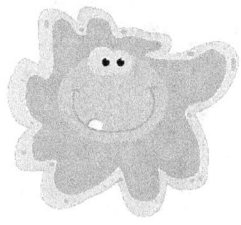 Eva, now toting a brand new immune system brought about by eating a banana, lamb cutlet, carrot, brisket casserole, orange, mushrooms, hazelnuts, and by enjoying a bit of sunbathing (without sun cream), continued on her long journey.

Soon she reached a T junction at the end of the road, this time with a sign pointing left that said 'Insect Kingdom' (creepy, crawly and conformist), and one pointing to the right that said 'Vertebrate Kingdom' (fishy, bony and individual).

"Hmmm, I like the sound of 'individual', I think that would suit someone like me" thought Eva, showing an early sign of pre-brain self-awareness.

Around 500 million years ago, the Animal Kingdom domain split in two 'bilateral' (meaning animals with a front and back) paths, one heading towards insects and the other heading towards vertebrates (animals with a backbone).

Eva continued down the 'backbone' road until she stumbled over a small shiny object. Having encountered something similar before (think baked beans), she knew how to tackle this one to get to the tasty contents...

Enter the Tinned Sardines

The sardine or pilchard refers to a small oily fish from the herring family. According to the UK Sea Fish Industry Authority, 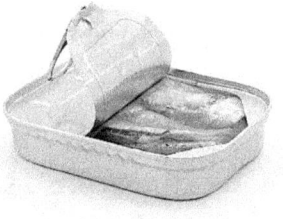 pilchards are larger sardines. There are many types of sardine, including the Rainbow sardine and the Goldstripe sardine. The one we are probably most familiar with is the young European pilchard.

The canning of sardines was originated by none other than Nicolas Appert (known as the "father of canning"). Mr Appert canned food to preserve it for Napoleon's soldiers to enjoy during the energy-sapping business of attempting to take over the world by force.

The tinned sardine has been described as the ultimate 'easily portable, non-perishable, self-contained food', which it certainly is - along with a whole lot more.

The canned sardine has an advantage over its fresh cousin by virtue of the way it is cooked. The tinned sardine breaks down, bones and all, and releases a nutrient that is a major building block for our bones and teeth, as well as contributing too many other vital processes.

The tinned sardine is also rich in another nutrient that is vital for bone formation - in fact it is required by every cell in our bodies, as Eva found out at the beginning of her journey in Chapter One.

The tinned sardine contains yet another nutrient that has a direct effect on bone health, a nutrient that Eva had previously got from a bit of sunbathing.

Eva gobbled down the sardines, including the soft bones, abandoning the tin (only advisable if you are near a recycling point!), and from the action of the minerals **Calcium** and

Phosphorus and the action of **Vitamin D** began to start feeling a little firmer.

*Calcium is a major building block in our bones, plays a vital role in the way our muscles work and is essential for good communication between our cells.

*Phosphorus is: an integral part of our bones, required by every cell in our bodies to work normally, critical in creating our energy, maintaining the chemical balance of our bodies.

*Vitamin D levels along with calcium levels have a direct effect on bone health.

*The **vEva** equivalents – Cheese, Muffins, Mushrooms*

With the beginnings of a skeleton and a newly formed tooth, Eva was still feeling absolutely famished and so went on in search of more food...

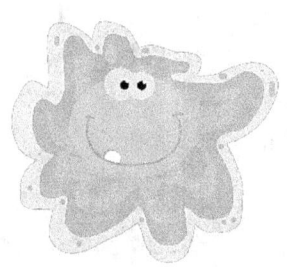

Bump! A large ferocious looking green and yellow bulbous spikey thing landed right in front of Eva. "Hey!" thought Eva, "Looks a bit weird, but could be scrumptious." And so she proceeded to chugalug the whole thing down...

Enter the Pineapple

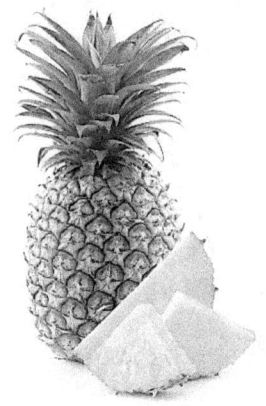

The pineapple was a favourite of the fierce Carib Indians (the tribe who gave their name to the Caribbean islands). This excellent fruit from Brazil and Paraguay was a staple of Indian feasts and was used to produce Indian wine. Due to the intense natural sweetness of the pineapple and the difficulty in cultivating it, it quickly became a fruit reserved for royalty.

The pineapple could therefore have been served as a dessert after the Anglo-Egyptian dish of swan and mushroom en croûte.

Along with its rich history, the pineapple boasts a nutrient that is vital for the creation of healthy bones and sinews. It also provides some important elements that Eva would have need of later, when she develops a brain and liver.

Having wolfed the whole pineapple down, Eva was now benefiting from the mineral **Manganese** and coming a little closer to a full set of bones.

*Manganese plays a role in detoxing our liver and brain and is important for the creation of healthy bone and sinew.

The next day, continuing down Backbone Road, Eva was still craving more of a certain nutrient to help complete her skeleton. Luckily, she spied a large red ball by the roadside...

Enter the Edam

Edam is a Dutch cheese that was the most popular cheese for 400 years, from the 14th to the 18th century. The name 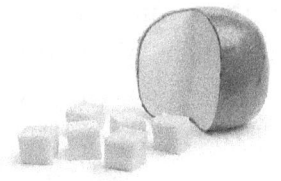 originates from the harbour of Edam, where most of this cheese was sold. Edam was a popular food on long sea voyages because of its ability to keep and age well.

It is said that in the early days of Edam production, this cheese was made using wooden forms that doubled as helmets, leading to the Dutch being nicknamed 'cheese heads'.

Modern Edam is made from pasteurised semi-skimmed milk, but Edam made from raw milk was revived in 2015.

The red-skinned Edam cheese contains more of a nutrient that is a major building block for our bones and teeth.

Eva dispatched the cheese, peel and all (must check the nutritional value of wax), and from the action of an additional dose of the mineral **Calcium** began to start feeling positively rigid.

*Calcium is so vital to our survival that low levels can result in the body extracting it from our bones to maintain the appropriate levels in the blood. We therefore need a daily intake of calcium for optimal health.

Eva now had enough bones to form a skeleton and needed to find something to fill up the newly formed space in her middle...

The skeleton

At birth, our skeleton is made up of 300 bones. As we grow, these fuse to form 206 bones. The longest bone in our body is the thigh bone or femur, with the smallest being the stirrup bone found in our ears. Our bones are constantly being worn down and our entire skeleton is replaced every 10 years or so.

A conversation between 2 mammals with very different sized skeletons.

Elephant says to a mouse; "Oh my, aren't you small!"

Mouse replies; "well, I have been quite ill recently!"

Summary

Nutrients critical to healthy bones, sinews and teeth

1. Calcium
2. Phosphorus
3. Vitamin D
4. Manganese

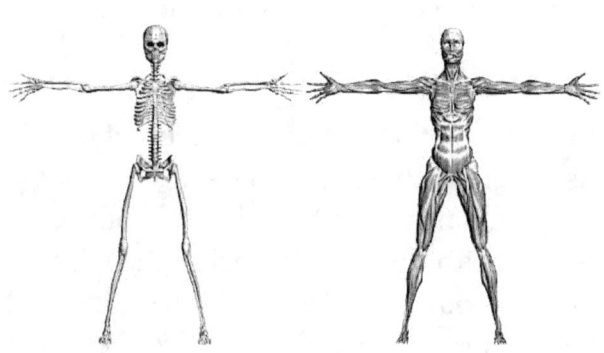

Chapter Four

The Heart and other Organs

"Only the pure in heart can make a good soup."
Ludwig van Beethoven

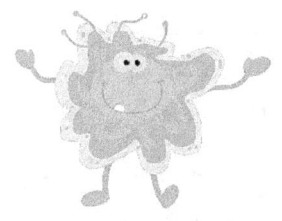 Eva - now transformed by a new skeleton and in possession of arms, legs and hair, all amazingly enabled by a tin of sardines (or cheese and muffins), a pineapple and a ball of Edam - found herself at another crossroads, with paths leading off in three directions.

Straight ahead was a signpost which said 'Boreo Kingdom' (perception, feelings and intelligence), the sign to her left said 'Laurasia Kingdom' (hoofs, humps and stripes), and on her right it said 'Marsupial Kingdom' (Australia).

"Hmmm, I like the sound of perception, feelings and intelligence..." thought Eva, showing signs of her desire for a conceptual framework to organise the ideas she was yet to have.

Around 60 to 150 million years ago, the Mammal vertebrates split into 3 distinct 'therian' or 'beast' categories: the Boreo therians went down the primate road, the Laurasian therians went down the horse, whale, camel, lion and dog road (amongst others), and the Marsupial therians went to Australia.

Eva set off down the primate road, thrilled at the possibilities the signposting hinted at - but first she needed some very specialised parts.

"What to eat next?" pondered Eva, and almost as soon as she had begun pondering, she stumbled over a white and pink lump lying right in the middle of primate road, "Yippee! More food!" thought Eva, and she quickly devoured this newly found treat.

Enter the Pork Belly

Pork bellies were first traded in the 'futures market' (risk management) in 1961 on the Chicago Exchange, and became an icon of futures trading, made even more iconic by the scene from the movie 'Trading Places'.

"Okay, pork belly prices have been dropping all morning, which means that everybody is waiting for it to hit rock bottom, so they can buy cheap and go long."
Billy Ray – Trading Places

The pork belly is very popular in Chinese cuisine and many other world cuisines, with the UK going for the slow roast gastro pub method of bringing back great *cheap* ingredients, and making them simply great ingredients.

The pork belly is packed with a 'bigger' nutrient vital to the development of cells, bones, and of course organs.

Having devoured the pork belly, Eva - fired up with a great amount of **Protein** - was now ready to begin developing some major protein-based parts of the body that carry out highly specialised functions.

*Protein is a vital macronutrient required as a component of all the cells and organs in our bodies, it also controls the rate at which the myriad of chemical conversions in our cells take place.

*The **vEva** equivalents – Cheese, Soya products*

Shortly after eating the pork belly, Eva felt a small thump in her chest area, followed by another thump, and then another, and then another....

Eva had of course developed a heart! "Wow!" *felt* Eva, (as yet unaware of the argument as to the origin of feelings). "This strange beating is making me hungry."

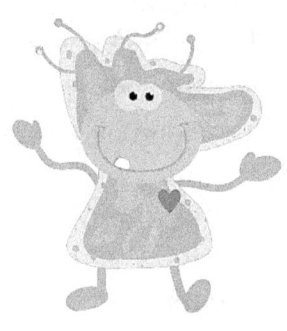

Excited by this new event, Eva saw a large white rock poking out from the grass verge at the edge of primate road. Eva immediately began licking it and was amazed at the tangy magical quality of the flavour.

Enter Salt- yes, Salt!

All life on our planet is dependent on salt, which comes either direct from the sea or is found in rock form.

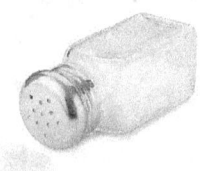

Salt has been used as currency since ancient times and is the origin of the word we have for being paid, as in 'salary'.

The 'wich' part of place names in the UK (such as Norwich) means a source of salt, and salt has been pivotal in the development of all civilisations.

Salt contains a nutrient that is vital to the correct functioning of the heart, along with playing a critical role in our absorption of **all** nutrients.

Having licked the rock of salt, Eva was now benefiting from the minerals **Sodium** and **Chloride,** and with her new-found heartbeat almost regular, she just needed another nutrient to complete this system.

Sodium and chloride are critical to the maintenance of heart function, muscle contraction, and the digestion and transport of nutrients into our cells.

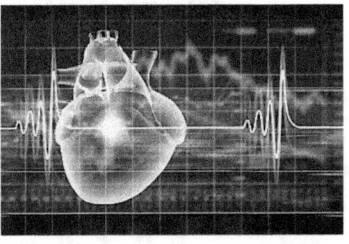

The dangers of salt debate

Much ink has been spilled and hefty words uttered about the dangers of salt. The latest study to emerge, involving 30,000 people, found that low-sodium intake is associated with more heart attacks, strokes, and deaths. The study also found that people with high blood pressure and high salt intake were at an increased risk of heart problems.

To maintain a healthy balance it is perhaps best to keep to the recommended daily amount (RDA), of around 5 grams.

N.B.: Much processed food has very high levels of refined salt added to make up for the abject lack of flavour, so always check the label.

Feeling pretty savoury, Eva moved further down primate road until she spotted a pile of muddy lumps. "These might be yummy," pondered Eva, whose thoughts such as they were tended to be guided by this sole principle.

Enter the Potato

In 1536, the Spanish Conquistadors (not generally known for their tolerant 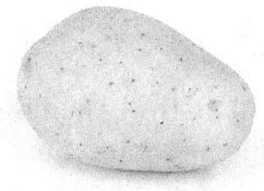 integration with native peoples) conquered Peru and discovered the potato.

Around 50 years later, Sir Walter Raleigh introduced potatoes to Ireland.

Potatoes are easier to cultivate than wheat and oats and - aided by the levels of nutrition they offer - took off as a new staple food.

In 1897 during the Alaskan gold rush, potatoes achieved the same value as gold as nutrition was in short supply, and as we all know wealth without health is of no use at all.

Along with much other goodness, potatoes possess a nutrient that, along with salt, maintains the balance of our heartbeat. This nutrient also plays a critical role in our absorption of **all** nutrients.

Eva gulped down the potato and 'regulated' her new heartbeat with the help of the mineral **Potassium.**

Potassium is critical to the maintenance of muscle contraction, heart function, and the transport of nutrients in and out of our cells.

What of potassium and the banana?

Traditionally, bananas have been considered to be high in potassium, with 330 mg per banana. This sounds like a lot until you compare it to the adult recommended daily amount (RDA) of 4,700 mg. This means that the banana (great as it is for other nutrients) only meets 8% of your RDA for potassium, whereas an average portion of cooked potatoes will meet 20% or more.

N.B. It is worth a mention here that keeping our salt intake in parity with our potassium intake is now recommended to maintain heart function and stable blood pressure.

With a new found thirst brought on by the salt, Eva had begun to develop a yearning for something to 'drink', but before a 'session' would be advisable, she needed another vital organ to be in top shape.

Now familiar with the goodies that the primate road was turning up, Eva set off in pursuit of - of course - her next meal. At this point, a small brown paper bag came rolling down the road and burst open, shedding tiny green, red and brown discs all over Eva's feet. "Aha!" thought Eva.

Enter the Lentils

Archaeologists have dated the origins of lentils to 13,000 years ago, in Greece. The Greeks were great lovers of 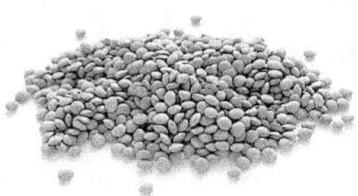 lentil soup, and the Greek satirical writer also referred to as the Father of Comedy, Aristophanes, is quoted as saying "You, who dare insult lentil soup, sweetest of delicacies."

One wonders who the "You" is referencing, perhaps the targets of Aristophanes' biting criticism of war profiteers.

Interestingly, Hippocrates is credited with prescribing lentil soup for liver complaints...

About Hippocrates

Hippocrates, who lived 2,500 years ago, is referred to as the 'father of modern medicine'. Modern medics take the 'Hippocratic Oath', which describes an ethical and moral code for the medical practitioner. Although this practice is no longer compulsory, it is still a symbolic part of many medical graduation ceremonies.

There is some controversy associated with the famous "let food be your medicine" quote being an accurate portrayal of Hippocrates' philosophy of medicine. Some academics attest that the real quote should be "let not thy food be confused with thy medicine". However, upon closer inspection of the surviving teachings surrounding Hippocrates, this could be said to amount to the same thing.

Hippocrates was at pains to point out that the wrong food eaten in the wrong way (raw, for example) caused problems that could be rectified by the right food eaten in the right way.

Perhaps a more accurate quote would be "let the right food eaten in the right way be your medicine". Either way, the guiding principle of food as medicine remains the same.

The amazing lentil contains several nutrients vital for the correct functioning of our livers.

Luckily for Eva, the bag of lentils had conveniently arrived ready cooked, and as Eva nibbled on these ancient favourites, she began to benefit from 4 nutrients.

The essential amino acid **Threonine,** the mineral **Manganese** (topping up the supply of this mineral she had earlier got from the pineapple), the newly classified nutrient **Choline**, and more of the **Pantothenic acid** (B5) she had gained from the broad beans in chapter 1.

*Threonine helps with liver function and prevents and corrects the accumulation of excess fat in the liver.

*Manganese plays a role in detoxing our liver.

*Choline has been shown to stop liver damage from fats and cholesterol.

*Pantothenic acid enables our liver to cope with toxins.

Now equipped with a strong and vital liver to go with her new heart, Eva went in search of something to slake her salty thirst and noticed a pile of fermenting red baubles...

Enter Red Wine

Evidence of wine production has been found as early as 8,000 years ago in Europe and has been celebrated as a ritualised drink ever since.

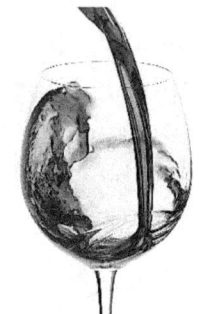

The earliest remains of a 'winery' were found in Armenia and date to about 6,000 years ago.

Wine features heavily in many world religions and mythologies (these two words being largely interchangeable).

Red wine is sometimes accredited as the reason for the 'French Paradox', i.e. the paradox of French people having a very low incidence of heart disease despite shovelling animal fats, cigarettes and vats of red wine down their discerning gullets. This phenomenon has confused scientists for many years, with animal fats and red wine now being looked at for their contribution to this conundrum.

In addition to its much appreciated intoxicating effects, red wine is an amazing source of organ-supporting nutrients.

Eva, needless to say, quaffed this fermented juice straight down and immediately started to benefit from the organ-enhancing minerals **Iron** and **Copper**, along with the protective power of the phytochemicals **Resveratrol** and **Flavonoids.** Eva was also benefiting from the product of fermentation known as **Alcohol**.

*Diets high in flavonoids lead to a considerable reduction in the risk of heart disease, stroke, high blood pressure, cancer, osteoporosis and cataracts and may be neuroprotective.

*In a test tube, Resveratrol has been shown to inhibit the development of several types of cancer and as an effective antioxidant.

*Many studies on disease occurrence in humans have shown that moderate alcohol consumption greatly reduces the risk of heart disease.

Eva - now a little tipsy, but with a fully functioning liver helping to process the alcohol, and plenty of ongoing support for her new-found organs - continued a little more jauntily down primate road. Eva was humming a tune as she went, when right in front of her appeared a jar of white pulp.

Now becoming familiar with packaging, Eva quickly worked out how to gain entry to the jar and swilled down the contents. "Tangy," thought Eva.

Enter the Sauerkraut

Sauerkraut is the
German word for
'sour cabbage' and
is salted and
fermented
cabbage.
The Roman

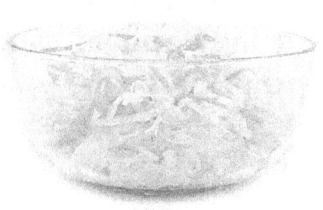

senator, Cato the Elder, who lived 2,200 years
ago and loved his agriculture, mentions
preserving cabbage in salt. Sauerkraut features
mainly in Eastern European and Germanic
cuisine but also appears in French and Dutch
cuisine.

Sauerkraut was used by ancient German
mariners on long voyages and provided just
enough vitamin C for them to avoid scurvy.

During WWI, due to concerns that the
American public would reject an ingredient
with a German name, sauerkraut was
temporarily renamed to 'Liberty Cabbage'. It is
ironic to note that the next time a food was
renamed in this way, it was to pass judgement
on a nation that *refused* to go to war. In 2003,
the US House of Representatives renamed the
'French fries' served in their canteens to

'freedom fries', as the French had opposed going to war with Iraq.

Having imbibed this tangy fermented victual, Eva gained some extra **Lactobacillus** (whose acquaintance she had first made at the bacteria and virus party), along with some other good bacteria. The natural bacteria or 'probiotics' in sauerkraut now added help to the system of moving food through Eva's gut and digesting nutrients.

The fermentation process sauerkraut undergoes creates lactic acid bacteria, including lactobacillus and pediococcus - bacteria that improve the digesting environment.

About digestion

As an amoeba, Eva had a very simple system of intracellular digestion, meaning that the food she ate entered a storage bubble in her single cell, whereupon enzymes are released to breakdown and digest the food. Now this system, whilst being effective, was not up to the job of dealing with her new-found diet of casseroles, cutlets, rice, oranges, tinned sardines and red wine. Eva urgently needed the help of some other single-cell organisms to aid her digestion.

Eva had met the bacteria lactobacillus at the party and developed 'gut flora', a complex community of

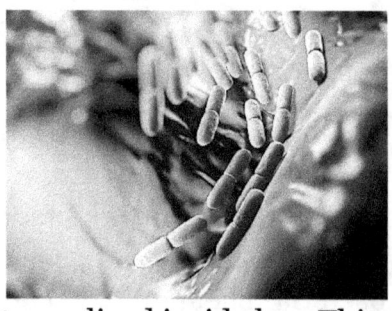

microorganisms that now lived inside her. This gut flora region is now referred to as our 'gut microbiome' and we also have a skin microbiome. Our overall microbiome is often referred to as the 'forgotten organ', as much research is now showing the pivotal importance of this system to our overall health (including mental health).

A microbiome – the microorganisms in a particular environment within the body.

A microorganism – an organism that can only be seen with a microscope and typically consists of a single-cell.

Interestingly, microbiologists estimate that there are 10 times as many bacterial cells as human cells in our body, giving an approximate total number of cells of 370 trillion!

Other good sources of digestion-aiding bacteria are yogurt and the Korean favourite of fermented cabbage known as Kimchi.

At this point, the constantly hungry Eva remembered she still had a half a can of baked beans from earlier and sat down to enjoy them once more.

Re-enter the Baked Beans

Baked beans contain another nutrient that maintains the health of our digestive system, specifically our bowels.

Baked beans are high in the nutrient **Fibre**.

Fibre is the indigestible part of a plant that - along with maintaining healthy bowels - also provides protection for our heart and arrests the development of diabetes.

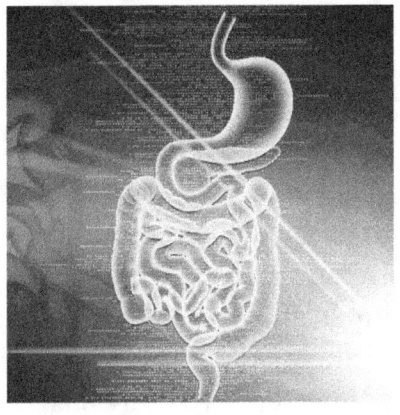

Fibre has also been shown to escort the antioxidant goodness of fruit and vegetables through to our colon. From here, these chemicals can be released and clean up our intestine environment, or enter our circulatory system for the cleansing and repairing activity our ongoing health requires.

Fibre maintains healthy bowels, protects against heart disease and strokes and arrests the development of diabetes.

Eva was now equipped with a stable beating heart, a clean liver and a powerful digestive system, along with a few others bits I haven't mentioned.

However, Eva knew she was still missing one other vital organ...

About organs

Like safaris, humans have what is known as the "Big Five". In the case of the safari, these are the lion, elephant, buffalo, leopard and rhino. In our case, these are the heart, liver, kidneys, lungs and skin. All these organs are made of 'protein' and their vital functioning is supported on a daily basis by many vitamins, minerals and phytochemicals.

Debate between organs as to who should be in charge of the body:

"I should be in charge," said the appendix, "Because I am removed from the function of the modern body and can therefore remain wholly objective and fair.

And if I don't get my way, I'll explode and kill us all!"

Summary

Nutrients critical to healthy organs

1. Protein
2. Salt
3. Potassium
4. Manganese
5. Threonine
6. Choline
7. Pantothenic acid (B5)
8. Iron
9. Copper
10. Phytochemicals
11. Fermented foods
12. Fibre
13. Alcohol (optional)

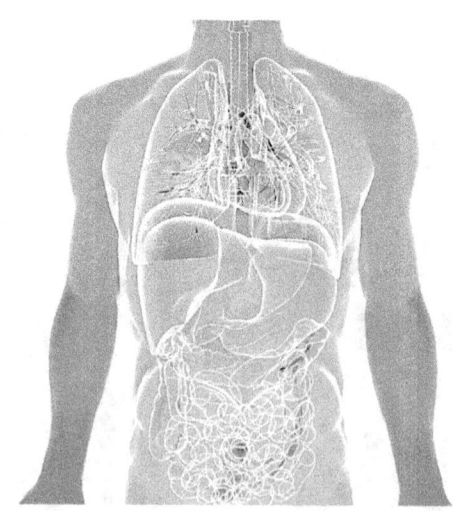

Chapter 5

The Brain

"The human brain has 100 billion neurons, each neuron connected to 10 thousand other neurons. Sitting on your shoulders is the most complicated object in the known universe."
Michio Kaku – Professor of Theoretical Physics

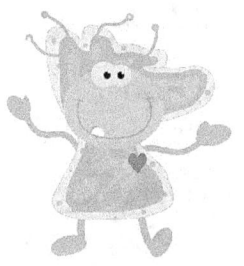

Eva, now with her 'big five' organs and a digestive system supported by pork belly (or cheese and tofu), salt, spuds, lentils, red wine, sauerkraut and beans, still needed one more major organ to continue her evolution.

Eva again found herself at a crossroads. To her left, there was a sign to the 'Neanderthal Kingdom' (extinction or hybridisation), to her right, a signpost said 'Denisovan Kingdom' (extinction or hybridisation) and straight ahead was a signpost marked 'Homo sapiens Kingdom' (space travel, the internet and smartphones).

"It has to be whatever space travel, the internet and smartphones means!" thought Eva.

Around 500,000 years ago, early humans went down 3 paths: the path of the Neanderthal, the Denisovan, and the Homo sapiens path. The Neanderthals and Denisovans were thought not to have survived, but Homo sapiens went on to become the modern human being. More current thinking attributes the modern human to potentially being a hybrid of all 3 paths.

Eva set off down Homo sapiens road, wondering what she would encounter next.

In the distance, she saw smoke billowing from a small hut. "Now I have to get me some of that action," thought Eva. Venturing inside the hut, Eva saw many brown oval-shaped objects hanging from the ceiling.

Enter the Kipper

Like all smoked food, the origin of the kipper is accredited to 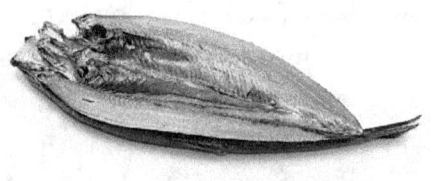 an "accident". According to folklore, a herring drying factory caught fire, and 'kippers' were discovered in the smouldering remains the next morning.

Great as that sounds, the more likely explanation is that the tradition of salting and smoking fish goes back millennia, and kippers are part of this heritage.

Kippers from the Isle of Man, Northumberland and Scotland are exported around the world, and to this day remain my dad's, (the son of the chicken's foot jelly toting Billingsgate fishmonger) favourite fish dish.

Like all oily fish and many white fish, kippers contain a nutrient that makes up close to 20% of our brains cerebral cortex, the part of our brain responsible for thought and action, plus another nutrient vital to our early brain development.

Eva couldn't resist this salty smoky treat and ingurgitated it greedily (what other way is there to ingurgitate?). Once consumed, the kipper gave Eva its **Omega 3,** and soon she began to develop more comprehensive thoughts and a reinforcement of her life's action so far: that of eating, eating, and eating some more. The **Iodine** in the kipper provided support for Eva's thyroid, which is central to our brain development, heart function and bone maintenance.

*Omega 3 EPA/DHA significantly reduces our risk of Alzheimer's, other forms of dementia, heart disease, and stroke.

*Iodine is critical to the early development of a baby's brain, so iodine levels are particularly important for pregnant and breast-feeding women.

*The **vEva** equivalents –Flaxseeds, Chia seeds, Rapeseed oil, Walnuts, Seaweed, Yogurt*

About the Omega 3s

There are 4 types of Omega 3: EPA, DHA and DPA from fish and meat sources, and ALA from both meat and vegetarian sources. The Omega 3 ALA we get from rapeseed oil, for example, has to be converted by us to the more powerful form of EPA/DHA.

Now enjoying a conceptual framework within which to organise her next course of action, Eva of course continued

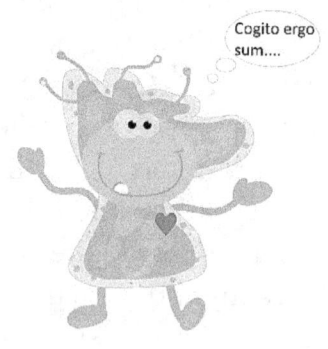

on her life's mission of discovering more food.

Bowling down Homo sapiens road with her new-found powers of thought, Eva spotted a small brown barrel-shaped novelty rolling towards her and coming to rest at her feet. "Boy, somebody up there likes me," thought Eva, her newly-found comprehension leading her into a traditional view of the relationship between us and the universe (as a starting point, hopefully).

Enter the jar of Peanut Butter

In 1890, an American chemist developed peanut paste as a source of nutrition for people who had 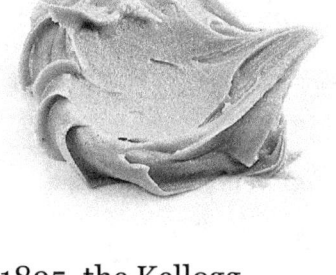 difficulty chewing. In 1895, the Kellogg brothers patented the peanut butter process involving boiling the nuts, which has now changed to roasting them.

It is estimated that around £550 million pounds worth of peanut butter are consumed in the US every year.

Médecins Sans Frontières (or 'Doctors Without Borders') hand out supplies of Plumpy'nut (a type of peanut butter) to malnourished children, with dramatic weight and health gaining results. A single pack contains 500 calories, can be stored unrefrigerated for 2 years, and requires no cooking or preparation.

Peanut butter contains a vital nutrient for our brain health and the health of our heart and skin.

Eva loved the taste of this creamy, crunchy substance and crammed so much in her mouth that she couldn't hum for a full 10 minutes. Eva had now received a good dose of **Omega 6** and was enjoying even greater clarity of thought, so she began pondering what she might find next.

*Omega 6 plays an important role in brain function, has been shown to enable our cells to communicate effectively, combat infection, regulate inflammation and promote blood clotting.

About the Omegas 3 and 6

Whilst the Omega 6 fatty acid is vital for human health, scientists have highlighted the problem of too much Omega 6, particularly in processed foods, leading to an imbalance between Omega 3 and Omega 6. These two fatty acids compete for absorption when there is too much Omega 6. This results in the health benefits being negated, and problems with unregulated inflammation can occur. Unregulated inflammation is a known starting point for several chronic disease states.

The current advice is to cut down on processed foods that use refined vegetable oils which are very high in Omega 6, and ensure a good supply of Omega 3.

With all the pondering, Eva was, of course, soon feeling hungry again. "What to eat now?" she thought.

With her newly developed cognisance, Eva remembered that she had some spinach left in her little pack and quickly sat down to finish it off.

Re-enter the Spinach

Unbeknownst to Eva, the spinach also contains some nutrients critical to brain health that work together in ways we do not yet fully 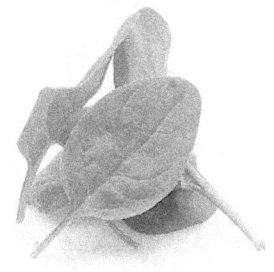 understand, to protect our cognitive ability.

Spinach (as we know from chapter one) contains **Folate** (B9), which is vital for healthy cell replication.

Folate is also essential for normal brain function and works with the **Vitamin K1** and the phytochemicals known as **Lutein** and **Beta Carotene** in spinach, to protect our awareness, knowledge, perception, recognition, appreciation and consciousness as we age.

Information from research carried out by the Rush University Medical Centre

The relationship between the liver and brain

Our liver naturally produces a steroid we know as **Cholesterol**.
Cholesterol is a vital component of every living cell of every living organism on earth and is vital for the functioning of the brain.

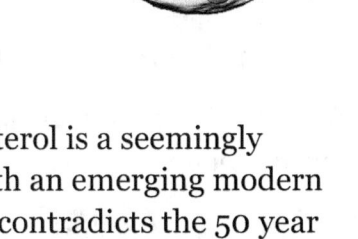

The subject of cholesterol is a seemingly controversial one, with an emerging modern view that completely contradicts the 50 year old concept of good and bad cholesterol levels, and the need to lower one's cholesterol levels.

There has been a lot of focus on the need to lower ones cholesterol levels, with various medications and fortified foods on offer to achieve just that.

Suffice it to say that a substance produced naturally by the liver that forms a vital part of our bodies' central mechanisms is highly likely to be 'good', and I will leave the argument there for now.

*Cholesterol is a natural steroid that is a vital component of every cell of every living organism on earth.

Sexist brain joke

An alien walked into a shop and told the owner that he came from Mars and wanted to buy a brain for research.

"How much is this one?" he asked.

"That one is a monkey brain, and its £20," the owner explained.

"How much is that one?" the alien asked.

"That one is a female brain, and it's £100," the owner replied.

"And how much is that one?" the alien asked.

"That one is a male's brain and it is £500" the owner explained.

"Why so expensive?" the alien asked.

The owner answered, "Well, it's hardly been used!"

Summary

Nutrients critical to brain health

1. Omega 3
2. Iodine
3. Omega 6
4. Folate
5. Vitamin K1
6. Lutein
7. Beta carotene
8. Cholesterol

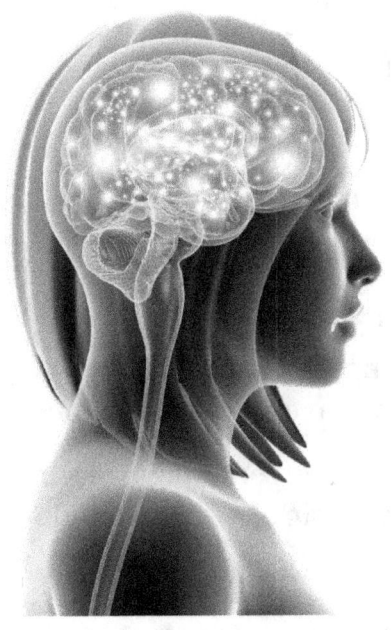

Chapter 6

The Final Ingredient

Eva had now completed her 3,500 million year journey from a single-cell amoeba down the evolutionary path to becoming a 37.2 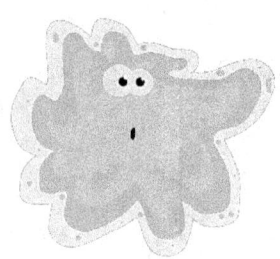 trillion cell, self-repairing and self-regulating, fully cognisant and self-aware human being (albeit with a somewhat unique appearance).

This was a journey only enabled by the food she encountered along the way, and there was one last ingredient she could benefit from to both complete 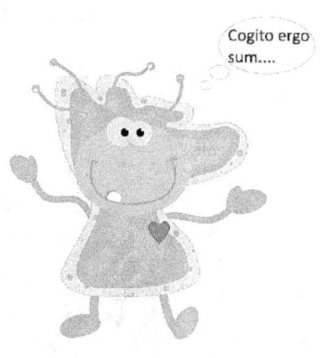 her journey and ensure her ongoing health.

"Hmmm... that green thing looks like broccoli", thought Eva, using her new-found recognition skills.

Enter the genius of Broccoli

Broccoli is a type of cabbage belonging to the mustard family. It is a fast growing plant that has been cultivated since ancient Roman times.

Broccoli was introduced to England around 1720 and has become a firm favourite vegetable accompaniment to arguably the greatest meal on Earth, the Roast Dinner.

Broccoli contains a whole host of nutrients that work together synergistically to provide an amazing array of benefits to the 37.2 trillion cells that make us up.

What's in broccoli?

Broccoli contains 12 **Vitamins**, 11 **Minerals**, all the **Essential Amino Acids** and the Phytochemicals known as **Flavonoids, Quercetin** and **Lutein**.

The nutrient synergies

The **Riboflavin** (B2) works with the **Thiamin** (B1) and the **Folate** as powerful protectors of DNA, ensuring health and preventing cancer.

The **Vitamin C** in broccoli enhances the absorption of the **Iron**, both powerful antioxidants (or cleansers and repairers) and vital for immune system, brain, blood and skin health.

The mineral **Selenium** regenerates the power of the **Vitamins E and C** for more powerful antioxidant activity and support for our skin and immune system.

The phytochemical **Lutein** interacts with the **Vitamin K1** and **Folate** to stave off cognitive decline by 12 years, as a recent study has shown.

The phytochemical **Quercetin** has been shown to block the growth of cancer cells and suppress the development of tumours.

Broccoli also contains a great ratio of **Omega 3** to **Omega 6,** working together for brain and heart health.

In addition to all the above, when broccoli is chewed it releases another set of phytochemicals known as **Isothiocyanates.** These chemicals have been shown in studies to inhibit the development of cancer and control inflammation.

Isothiocyanates have also been specifically shown to enhance the genes associated with cancer prevention.

To cap all this, broccoli also contains good amounts of a compound known as **Alpha-Lipoic Acid.**

At Oregon State University (the world's leading centre for micronutrient science), researchers believe that lipoic acid kick-starts cells to regain the functions they naturally had in youth.

What this means is that as we regenerate, our new cells are younger than the ones expiring, affecting the rate at which we age.

Dr Royal Lee and Nutrient Synergy

Born in 1895, Dr Lee adopted an approach to nutrition that integrated science, agriculture, physiology, engineering, invention, politics, education, business, biochemical manufacturing, and philosophy.

The quote below sums up his approach to the synergy of nutrients.

"A vitamin as it appears in nature is never a single chemical, but rather it is a group of interdependent compounds that form a 'nutrient complex' so intricate that only a living cell can create it. And just as no single component of a watch keeps time, no single compound in a vitamin complex accounts for the vitamin's nutritive effect in the body. Only through whole, unprocessed foods can the synergistic effect of a true vitamin be delivered."

Dr Royal Lee - Also referred to as the "Einstein of nutrition"

Broccoli and evolution

Broccoli is just one example of the *exact* match that nature provides in ingredients to our development and ongoing health.

This small green plant provides support for:

Our incredibly precise **Immune System**

Our amazing **Blood**

The astonishing intricacy of our **Digestive System**

The most complex object in the known universe, our **Brain**

Our biggest organ, the **Skin**

Our phenomenal regenerating **Skeleton**

The billions of miles of **DNA** we have in our cells

The 2.5 billion **Heartbeats** we have in a lifetime

Our detoxifying, energy-creating **Liver**

And has anti-cancer and anti-ageing qualities...

At least that is what over 120 years of science tells us!

Eva carefully chewed and then swallowed the broccoli and sat down to put her feet up, secure in the knowledge that for now, her ongoing health was in good hands...

Almost the END

And so our little excursion with Eva into evolution, food and health comes to an end. I hope that, just like me, you are excited about your next meal, and the one after that, and the one after that...

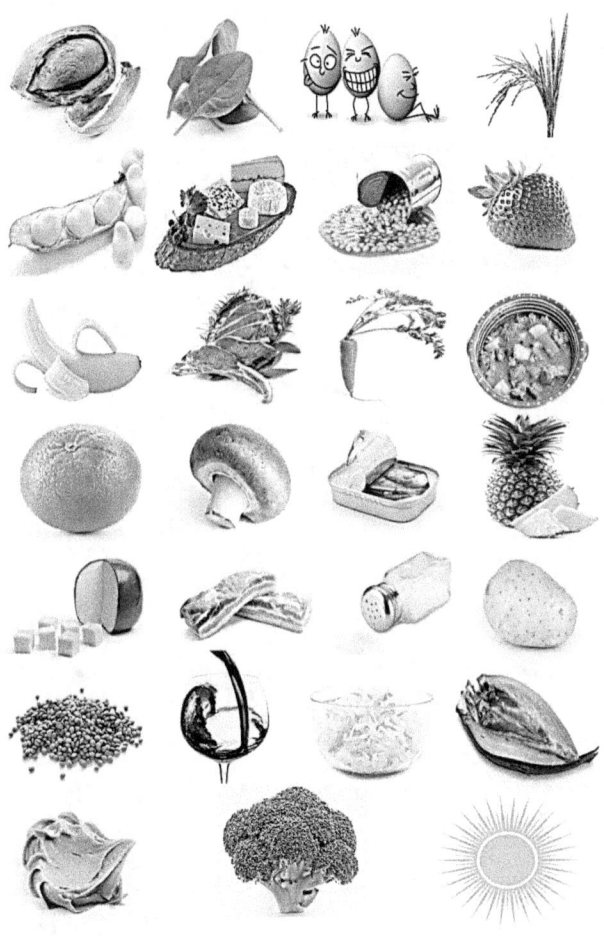

Conclusion

"Food is not just a source of energy or calories. Food is information. It contains instructions that affect every biological function of your body. It is the stuff that controls everything."
Dr Mark Hyman – Eat Fat Get Thin

The 5 Way Juxtaposition

The secret to maximising the 'information' and 'instructions' in food is knowing which nutrients are in which foods (**food composition data**), the health benefits of those nutrients (**the science**), how much we need on a daily basis (**RDAs**), the effects of cooking on nutrients (**retention factors**), and a comparison of the nutritional value of ingredients based on **realistic portion sizes**.

Which is why we have created an 'engine' to do all this for you.

Using all the incredible research, analysis and science that has been done and is ongoing, we can work with our 37.2 trillion cells to enhance our health and wellbeing, the health and wellbeing of our families, and the health and wellbeing of our clients.

Welcome to checkyourfood.com

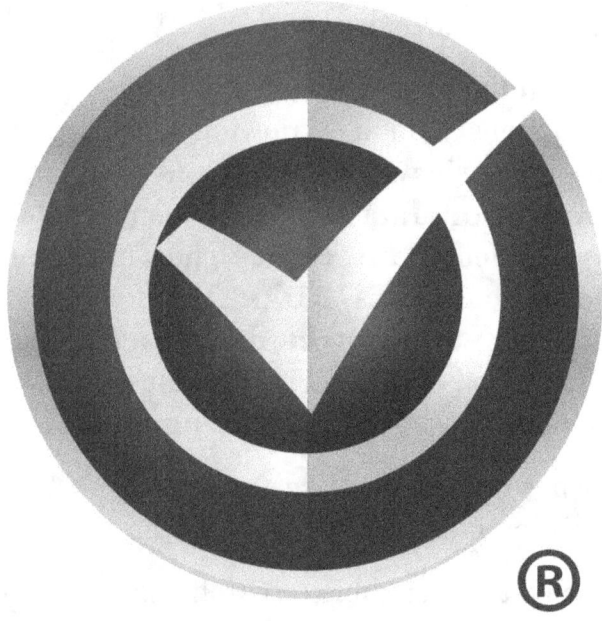

"Homo sum humani a me nihil alienum puto."

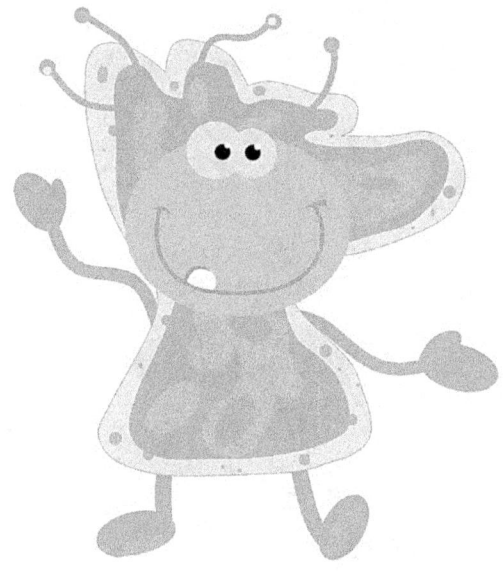

"I am a human being; nothing human is strange to me."

Bye from Eva

Starring Characters

Data, information and artwork sources

Checkyourfood.com (*science summaries*, nutrient amounts and the 5 Way Juxtaposition)

The Linus Pauling Institute – Oregon State University (science)

The National Academy of Sciences (RDA's)

The Rush University Medical Centre (greens and cognitive decline study)

The UK Institute of Food Research (food composition data)

The US Department of Agriculture (food composition data & cooking retention factors)

The National Centre for Biotechnology Information (science)

The Health Sciences Academy (science)

The Science Daily (science)

Wikipedia (history)

Matt Baker - Evolution and Classification of Life chart

dvarg – front cover image

Watchara Khamphonsaeng - rear cover image

The Author

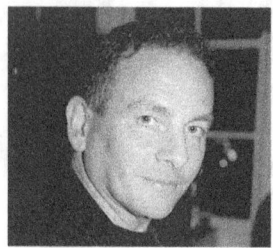

Matt Wright is the founder of checkyourfood.com, a researcher, an information systems expert, and above all a nutrient monomaniac.